ICS 11.020

SCM

世界中医药学会联合会
World Federation of Chinese Medicine Societies

SCM 52—2020

中药处方、调剂、给付与煎服要求
第1部分：中药处方要求

Requirements for Prescription, Dispensing, Delivery,
Decocting and Taking of Chinese Medicine
Part 1: Requirements for Prescription of Chinese Medicine

世界中联国际组织标准　　2020-7-2发布实施
International Standard of WFCMS　　**Issued & implemented on July 2, 2020**

中医古籍出版社
Publishing House of Ancient Chinese Medical Books

图书在版编目（CIP）数据

中药处方、调剂、给付与煎服要求 . 第 1 部分，中药处方要求：汉英对照 / 世界中医药学会联合会著 .— 北京：中医古籍出版社，2024.5
ISBN 978-7-5152-2452-7

Ⅰ . ①中… Ⅱ . ①世… Ⅲ . ①中药材—处方—汉、英 Ⅳ . ① R28

中国版本图书馆 CIP 数据核字（2022）第 011866 号

中药处方、调剂、给付与煎服要求　第 1 部分：中药处方要求

世界中医药学会联合会　著

责任编辑　张　楚
封面设计　艺点锦秀
出版发行　中医古籍出版社
社　　址　北京市东城区东直门内南小街 16 号（100700）
电　　话　010-64089446（总编室）010-64002949（发行部）
网　　址　www.zhongyiguji.com.cn
印　　刷　北京市泰锐印刷有限责任公司
开　　本　880mm×1230mm　1/16
印　　张　2.5
字　　数　85 千字
版　　次　2024 年 5 月第 1 版　2024 年 5 月第 1 次印刷
书　　号　ISBN 978-7-5152-2452-7
定　　价　36.00 元

目　　次
Contents

前　言

请注意本文件的某些内容可能涉及专利。本文件的发布机构不承担识别专利的责任。

本文件《中药处方、调剂、给付与煎服要求》分为4个部分：

——第1部分：中药处方要求；

——第2部分：中药调剂要求；

——第3部分：中药给付要求；

——第4部分：中药煎服要求。

本部分为第1部分：中药处方要求。

主要起草单位：江西中医药大学、香港浸会大学、江西省中医药管理局、深圳市卫生健康发展研究和数据管理中心、澳门科技大学、深圳市卫生健康委员会、深圳市中医院、深圳市罗湖区中医院、深圳市人民医院、深圳市标准技术研究院、深圳技术大学、中国人民解放军总医院第五医学中心、深圳统标科技有限公司、中国中医科学院中医药信息研究所、中国中药控股有限公司、中国食品药品检定研究院中药民族药检定所、美国杏林健康科技有限公司、澳洲全国中医药针灸学会联合会、澳大利亚澳华中医学会、澳大利亚中医药学会。

参与起草单位：北京中医药大学深圳医院（龙岗）、安徽广印堂中药股份有限公司、北京中医药大学东方医院、北京中医药大学东直门医院、亳州市永刚饮片厂有限公司、广东食品药品职业学院、汕头市澄海区中医医院、德国汉堡大学汉萨美安中医中心、广州市黄埔区穗东街夏园社区卫生服务站、广州市健桥惠泽有限公司、韩国庆熙大学、加拿大中医学院、江西江中中药饮片有限公司、江西省药品检验检测研究院、加州中医药大学、美国金禾中医药有限公司、纽约中医学院、南方医科大学深圳医院、汕头大学医学院第二附属医院、汕头市澄海区人民医院、汕头市澄海区溪南镇卫生院、汕头市中心医院、汕头市中医医院、上海中医药大学、深圳市华辉药业有限公司、深圳市药品检验研究院、深圳市中医药企业标准联盟、深圳市中医药学会、首都医科大学附属北京地坛医院、苏州信亨自动化科技有限公司、中山市中医院。

主要起草人：廖利平、吕爱平（中国香港）、肖小河、吴培凯、李顺民、曾庆明、邓雪枝、兰青山、马双成、赵永红、周华、徐子渠、石燕红、刘希伟、陈明人、左铮云、杨明、周平生、李海燕、杨具荣、李锦轩、林子强（澳大利亚）、姚克勤、张翼（澳大利亚）、朱丽华、程晗、郑建华（澳大利亚）、梁葆山（美国）。

参与起草人及审阅专家（按姓氏拼音排序）：蔡本辉、蔡楚喜、蔡沛彪、蔡文伟、蔡晓纯、蔡永江、陈健星、陈洁、陈镍、陈权韩、谌瑞林、陈思远、陈玩珊、陈业孟（美国）、程仕萍、丛佳林、崔欣羽、丁演龄、杜建强、高广印、高新颜、龚千锋、古旭明、关志宇、郭晓秋、何杜朋、何浪、胡世平、胡小婕、胡新华、华国栋、黄剑帆、黄举凯、黄展辉、简晖、赖满香、李静、李锐键、李咏、梁晖宙（美国）、林韩、林明欣、林树旭、刘宝河、刘炽京（澳大利亚）、刘荣华、刘勇、路海英、罗光明、穆风杨、彭映梅、史花兰、王伽伯、王淑红、王伟群、王越、肖雪青、许素文、许晓瑜、许妍、薛春苗、Yang Woongmo（韩国）、杨西晓、杨晓晖、杨银芳、叶年华、易炳学、余沐珍、余亚薇、袁晓宁（加拿大）、原文鹏、Ron Zaidman（美国）、曾长龙、查青林、章德林、张金莲、张力、张萍、张寿文、章文春、赵恒伯、赵文静、赵振萍（美国）、朱卫丰、邹健生。

本文件的起草程序遵守了世界中医药学会联合会发布的《世界中医药学会联合会国际组织标准管理办法》和 SCM 0001–2009《标准制定和发布工作规范》。

引　言

中医药是中华民族的文化瑰宝。中医诊疗服务过程，从病人就诊开始，到医生辨证论治，开具正确的中药处方，再到中药的调剂，各个环节中均有相应关键节点：中医师如何在辨证论治的指导下遣方用药；药房和中药处方如何管理；药事人员如何合规地审方，如何正确地调剂，即中药饮片的给付 / 配方；患者如何自行选购合格的中药饮片进行准确配方和合理煎煮；病人又如何正确服用中药。以上的每一个环节和流程，呈现分散状态，没有形成有机结合，影响中药用药安全与有效，损害消费者切身权益，进而降低中医药服务质量和声誉。

因此，有必要将分散的中药服务环节和流程整合成为一个完整的体系，以标准的形式固化下来，构建一个质量可以追溯的中药服务流程，进而达到减少医疗差错，改善医患关系，避免医疗事故，提高医疗服务水平，保障人民用药安全与有效，维护消费者合法权益的目的。

《中药处方、调剂、给付与煎服要求》旨在整合中医药服务流程，建立、健全中医药标准服务体系与认证制度，规范行业行为和药事人员职业操守，营造中药种植、生产、流通、用药的安全与有效，促进中药贸易公平、公正、和谐和科学发展的良好氛围，让世界各国人民共享中医药发展成果，为全人类的健康作出应有的贡献。

本文件为《中药处方、调剂、给付与煎服要求》第 1 部分，规范了开具中药处方的要求。它与第 2、3、4 部分形成无缝对接。医生开具中药处方是医疗活动的重要组成部分，是非常严肃和严谨的行为，是整个中药药事服务流程的首要工作、重中之重。

中药处方、调剂、给付与煎服要求 第 1 部分：中药处方要求

1 范围

本文件规定了中药处方的总体要求、内容和书写要求。同时，对中药处方权资格、贵重药品处方、毒性药品、麻醉药品处方和协定处方的管理等进行了规范。

本文件适用于与处方开具、调剂、保管相关的医疗机构及其人员。

2 规范性引用文件

下列文件中的内容通过文中的规范性引用而构成本文件必不可少的条款。其中，注日期的引用文件，仅该日期对应的版本适用于本文件；不注日期的引用文件，其最新版本（包括所有的修改单）适用于本文件。

GB/T 7027 信息分类和编码的基本原则与方法

GB/T 7635.1 全国主要产品分类与代码　第 1 部分：可运输产品

GB 12904 商品条码　零售商品编码与条码表示

GB/T 17710 信息技术　安全技术　校验字符系统

GB/T 31773 中药方剂编码规则及编码

GB/T 31774 中药编码规则及编码

GB/T 31775 中药在供应链管理中的编码与表示

ISO 18662–1 *Traditional Chinese Medicine—Vocabulary—Part 1: Chinese Materia Medica*

ISO 18662–2 *Traditional Chinese Medicine—Vocabulary—Part 2: Processing of Chinese Materia Medica*

ISO 18668–1:2016 *Coding System for Chinese Medicines—Part 1: Coding Rules for Chinese Medicines*

ISO 18668–2:2017 *Coding System for Chinese Medicines—Part 2: Codes for Decoction Pieces*

ISO 18668–3:2017 *Coding System for Chinese Medicines—Part 3: Codes for Chinese Materia Medica*

ISO 18668–4:2017 *Coding System for Chinese Medicines—Part 4: Codes for Granule Forms of Individual Medicinals for Prescriptions*

ISO 20333:2017 *Coding Rules for Chinese Medicines in Supply Chain Management*

ISO 20334:2018 *Coding System of Formulae*

3 术语和定义

下列术语和定义适用于本文件。

3.1
中医师

具备中医学专业知识，依法取得当地卫生、医药部门或者行业管理部门认可的执业资质或要求，在医疗、预防、保健机构中执业的专业人员。

3.2
中药师

具备中药学专业知识，依法取得当地卫生、医药部门或者行业管理部门认可的执业资质或要求，在医疗、预防、保健机构中执业的专业人员。

3.3
医嘱

医生在医疗活动中根据病人的病情和治疗的需要，对病人在用药、化验、饮食等方面的指示。

注 1：医嘱按照时效性分为长期医嘱和临时医嘱。长期医嘱指有效时间 24 小时以上，每日重复执行，医师注明停止时间后失效。长期备用医嘱是一种特殊长期医嘱，每执行一次需要在临时医嘱中进行相关记录。临时医嘱指有效时间 24 小时以内，执行完毕后失效。

注 2：医嘱按照内容分为用药医嘱、诊疗医嘱、护理医嘱、嘱托医嘱和特殊医嘱。本文件是指用药医嘱，是中药师审核、调配、核对，并作为患者用药凭证的医疗文书。

3.4
中药处方

由取得执业资格的医生（又称为“医师”）在诊疗活动中为患者开具的，载有中药药品名称、数量、煎服方法等内容和任何一种制剂的制备，供中药专业技术人员审核、调配、核对，并作为发药凭证的医疗用药的医疗文书。

注 1：中药处方又称处方 / 药方，既是医师给中药调剂人员的书面通知 / 医嘱，又是中药调剂工作的依据，也是计价、统计的凭证，具有法律上、技术上和经济上的意义。

注 2：中药处方是医师辨证论治的书面记录和凭证，反映了医师的辨证理法和用药要求。

3.5
协定处方

由医师、药师双方根据治疗需要协商确定并经医疗机构批准的本医疗机构常规处方，旨在用一组固定的药物处理某个常见的带共性的临床问题。

3.6
辨证论治

中医师根据患者的症状和体征，通过分析、综合，辨清疾病的病因、性质、部位和邪正之间的关系，概括、判断为某种病症，确定相应的治疗方法。

注 1：医生对疾病进行辨证诊断，是中医诊断应有的、特殊的内容，它是理法处方的主要依据，是中医认识和治疗疾病的基本原则，是中医学对疾病的一种特殊的研究和处理方法，也是中医学的基本特点之一。

注 2：证，是机体在疾病发展过程中的某一阶段的病理概括。它包括病位、病因、病性以及正邪关系，反映出疾病发展过程中某一阶段的病理变化的本质，因而它比症状更全面、更深刻、更正确地揭示了疾病的本质，比如，肝阳上亢、湿热下注。另一个需要明确的概念是“症”，比如发热、头痛、舌苔黄、脉数。

注 3： 辨证，是将四诊（望、闻、问、切）所收集的资料、症状和体征，通过分析、综合，辨清疾病的病因、性质、部位和邪正之间的关系，概括、判断为某种证。

注 4： 论治，是根据辨证的结果，确定相应的治疗方法。中医治病首先着眼于证，而不是病的异同。因此，同一疾病的不同证候，治疗方法就不同；而不同疾病，只要证候相同，便可以用同一方法治疗。这就是“同病异治、异病同治”。这种针对疾病发展过程中不同质的矛盾，用不同的方法去解决的法则，就是辨证论治的精神实质。

注 5： 辨证论治，是根据患者的不同症状，将其辨别为中医的不同证，加以灵活诊治。辨证论治要求医生把握动态的宇宙天气、动态的人、动态的疾病，运用中医天人合一学说，因时、因地、因人制宜，进行辨证论治，准确地把握人体与天地间的最佳平衡点，巧妙调节人体阴阳平衡，最终化疾病于无形。因为中医的灵活性、创造性，只要正确掌握辨证论治，即使没有明确的病名诊断，也能对这些疾病进行治疗。所以已知和未知的疾病，只要有症状，均可制订出诊疗方案，及时治疗，这正是中医学的最大特色之一。

注 6： 临床常用的辨证方法分为八纲辨证、气血津液辨证、脏腑辨证、六经辨证、卫气营血辨证、三焦辨证、经络辨证。这些方法各有特色，在临床诊断病例上，医生可以灵活选用或者整合以上方法进行辨证论治。

3.7
毒性

中药对人体的有害性。

4 总体要求

4.1 处方权的取得

获得执业资格，在当地医疗卫生主管部门注册，并被医疗机构聘用者，具有该机构处方权资格。

4.2 处方的开具

4.2.1 中医师应根据医疗、预防、保健需要，按照诊疗规范、药品说明书的功效主治或适应证、药理作用、用法用量、禁忌、不良反应和注意事项等，同时遵循辨证论治的原则开具处方。

4.2.2 危急状态下开具麻醉药品处方时，应使用淡红色麻醉药处方，并在处方右上角醒目位置标注“急”或“危急”，作为进入药品调剂“生命绿色通道”的提示。

4.2.3 开具儿科急诊处方时，医生应权衡第一实际需要选择色标处方：如果当时用药急迫性需要大于用药安全性需要，则采用淡黄色急诊处方；如果当时用药安全性需要大于用药急迫性需要，则采用淡绿色儿科处方。

4.3 处方的色标

为了增强医师、药师的视觉警觉意识，防止用药失误，确保用药安全，将处方分 4 种颜色，并在处方右上角标明处方色标。各类处方的颜色要求如下：

a）麻醉药品处方为淡红色；

b）急诊处方为淡黄色；

c）儿科处方为淡绿色；

d）普通处方为白色。

4.4 处方的时效性

为了保证临床用药的及时与有效，应保证处方的时效性。

中药处方开具当日有效。特殊情况下需延长有效期的，应由开具处方的医师注明有效期限，但有效期最长不应超过 3 天。

4.5 处方的修改

处方应字迹清楚，不应涂改。如需修改，应在修改处签名并注明修改日期。

4.6 处方的保存和销毁

处方由调剂处方的医疗机构妥善保存。各类处方的具体保存期限应遵守本国或本地区行业管理要求。

处方保存期满后，经医疗机构主要负责人批准后，整理、登记备案后，方可销毁。

4.7 其他要求

中药处方中所涉及的中药饮片应符合《濒危野生动植物种国际贸易公约》（CITES）的要求。

5 中药处方内容及书写要求

5.1 中药处方内容

应对处方书写的前记、正文和后记等内容与要求进行规范；应遵循安全、有效、经济的原则。

——处方前记，包括医疗、预防、保健机构名称，处方编号，费别，患者姓名、性别、年龄、门诊或住院病历号，科别或病室和床位号，临床诊断 / 中医诊断包括病名和证型（病名不明确的可不写病名），开具日期等。

——处方正文，以 Rp 或 R（拉丁文 Recipe“请取”的缩写）标示，饮片包括处方饮片名称、剂量剂数、用法；中成药处方应分列药品名称、规格、数量、用法用量。

——处方后记，包括医师签名和 / 或加盖专用签章，根据实际情况可添列特殊要求的项目，如价格、药品金额，以及审核、调配、核对、发药的药学专业技术人员签名和 / 或加盖专用签章。

5.2 中药处方书写要求

处方的书写要求应按处方前记、正文、后记的内容进行书写，同时应符合以下几个方面：

——应体现辨证论治、理法方药及其“君、臣、佐、使”的特点要求；

——中药饮片名称以当地官方语言书写，同时以拼音或拼音加拉丁文的形式进行备注；

——剂量使用法定剂量单位，用阿拉伯数字书写，原则上应以克（g）为单位，“g”（单位名称）紧随数值后；

——调剂、煎煮的特殊要求注明在药品名称右上方，并加括号，如打碎、先煎、后下等；

——对中药饮片的产地、炮制有特殊要求的，应在药品名称之前写明；

——根据整张处方药味多少选择每行排列的药味数，原则上要求横排且上下排列整齐；

——中药饮片用法用量应符合本国或本地区药典及行业管理规定，且无配伍禁忌。有超剂量使用和配伍禁忌时，应在药品名称上方再次签名；

——中药饮片剂数应以“剂”为单位；

——处方用法用量紧随剂数之后，包括每日剂量、采用剂型（水煎煮、酒泡、打粉、制丸、装胶囊等）、每剂分几次服用、用药方法（内服、外用等）、服用要求（温服、凉服、顿服、慢服、饭前服、饭后服、空腹服等）等内容；

示例：“每日 1 剂，水煎 400 mL，分早晚两次空腹温服”。

——按毒麻药品管理的中药饮片的使用应严格遵守有关法律、法规和规章的规定。

——严格遵守本国或本地区医疗卫生监管部门对某些中药饮片禁用或限制使用的相关规定。

5.3 中成药处方书写要求

——根据中医诊断（包括病名和证型）结果，辨证或辨证辨病结合选用适宜的中成药；

——中成药名称应使用经药品监督管理部门批准并公布的药品通用名称，院内中药制剂名称应使用经省级药品监督管理部门批准的名称；

——用法用量应按照药品说明书规定的常规用法用量使用，特殊情况需要超剂量使用时，应注明原因并再次签名；

——片剂、丸剂、胶囊剂、颗粒剂分别以片、丸、粒、袋为单位，软膏剂及乳膏剂以支、盒为单位，溶液制剂、注射剂以支、瓶为单位，应注明剂量；

——每张处方不应超过 5 种药品，每一种药品应分行顶格书写，药性峻烈的或含毒性成分的药物应避免重复使用，功能主治相同或基本相同中成药、含相同毒性药材中成药不宜叠加使用；

——中药注射剂应单独开具处方；

——中药处方的书写格式宜与电子病历相一致。

5.4 中药处方书写示例

中药饮片处方书写示例和中成药处方书写示例见附录 A。

6 中药处方权、处方调剂资格的管理

6.1 中药处方权的管理

6.1.1 留样备查

有处方权和临时处方权的医师签名式样和印模应在药学部门留样备案，医师不可擅自更改签名式样。医师需更改签名式样应重新登记留样备案。

6.1.2 中药麻醉药品处方权

医疗机构应按照本国或本地区卫生管理部门的规定，对本机构执业医师进行有关中药麻醉药品使用知识的培训、考核，经考核合格的，授予麻醉药品处方资格。执业医师取得麻醉药品处方资格后，方可在本医疗机构开具麻醉药品处方，但不应为自己开具该类处方。

6.1.3 处方的修改

医师开具的处方，各项目不应涂改，如需修改，应该在修改内容上划一道直线，修改前的内容

应该仍清晰可见，并在修改处重新签署姓名与修改日期。

中药学人员不应擅自修改医师处方，如遇缺药或处方错误等特殊情况需修改处方时，要退回医师修改签字后才能调配。

6.1.4　处方权的取消

医师被责令暂停执业、被责令离岗培训期间或被注销、吊销执业证书后，其处方权即被取消。

6.2　处方调剂资格的管理

6.2.1　处方调剂资格

取得中药学专业技术资格并符合本国或本地区的相关要求，并被用人机构聘用者，具有该机构处方调剂资格。

6.2.2　处方调剂资格的获取

满足处方调配资格要求的中药学人员应经用人单位考核，通过后才能获取处方调剂资格。

从事处方审核的技术人员应取得相关专业技术职务任职资格，并符合本国或本地区的相关要求。

6.2.3　留样备查

中药处方调剂人员签名式样应在本机构留样备查。

6.2.4　权限

中药学调剂人员有权监督、审核处方，参与临床合理用药。凡不符合规定的处方，有权拒绝调剂。

7　贵重药品的处方管理

7.1　贵重药品的分类和品种

贵重药品分为一类贵重中药和二类贵重中药。

纳入一类贵重中药管理的中成药和二类贵重中药管理的中药饮片品种，根据《贵重药品管理制度》和各药房实际情况选定。

7.2　一类贵重中药处方的管理

一类贵重中药应由专人专锁专账管理。一类贵重中药处方应单独开具，并单独合订存放。

8　协定处方管理

8.1　协定处方的制定原则

协定处方的制定原则应满足：

——必要性：确有必要用一组固定的药物处理某个常见的带共性的临床问题；
——合理性：应选择合理的药物，即应安全、有效、经济、合适；
——稳定性：因为协定处方的固体口服制剂在预先集中调配时，药物要暴露在空气中，且调配好的药物需要在简易包装中存放一定时间，故要求药物在空气中有较好的稳定性；
——协同性：处方各种药物之间没有配伍禁忌，最好能起减毒增效的作用。

8.2 协定处方的管理

8.2.1 协定处方的备案

协定处方应经本机构药事管理委员会审核同意并备案。

8.2.2 协定处方的使用

依据协定处方调配的药品及中药饮片代煎剂不应冠以成药名称或代号，开具协定处方（包括病历中书写协定处方）应书写组成处方的各具体药品名称；协定处方按照中药饮片处方格式书写。

协定处方不限制医师的灵活用药，可根据病情需要在协定处方的基础上加用药物，但不能减用协定处方的药物。

8.2.3 协定处方配药室的仪器要求

协定处方配药室应配备恒温恒湿仪器、净化设备或无菌工作台。配药室应定期消毒，工作环境整洁、无污染，注意防虫、防尘。所有配药工具都应定期消毒，防止药物污染。直接接触药品的包装材料应符合国家有关规定。

8.2.4 批量调配协定处方的记录

批量调配协定处方应有记录，记录中应注明调配日期，处方中药品的品名、规格，原包装的生产企业、批号、有效期，原包装药品数量和调配药品的数量，调配人、复核人应签名。

协定处方的包装袋上应贴有标签，注明处方药品通用名称、规格、数量、生产企业、批号、有效期的标签。

8.2.5 拆零用于协定处方调配的药品的使用

——拆零用于协定处方调配的药品应按品种、批号分批使用，拆零时注明拆零日期。
——拆零以后的药品，应采用原包装贮存。如采用其他容器贮存，直接接触药品的容器应符合药用包装要求和药品贮存要求，并应贴有药品通用名称、规格、生产企业、批号、有效期的标签。
——定期对拆零后储存在容器内的药品进行检查，发现有污染、变质和过期失效的药品应按规定及时处理。

9 麻醉药品和毒性药品处方要求

麻醉药品和毒性药品专用处方要求应严格遵守本国或本地区卫生管理部门相应规定，可参见附录B。

附录 A
（规范性）
中医医院中药处方样式和书写示例

中医医院中药饮片处方书写示例和中成药处方书写示例见图 A.1。

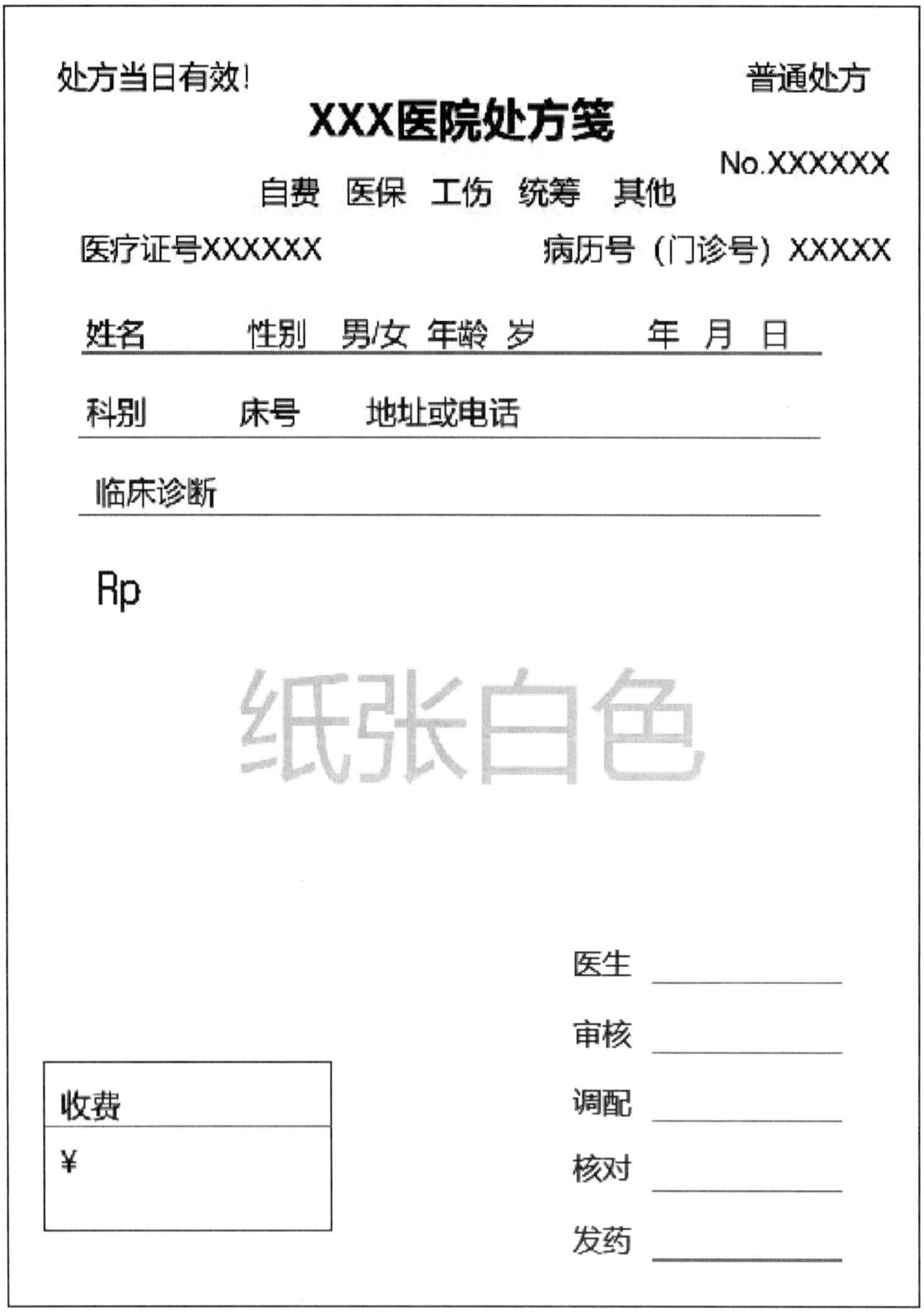

处方当日有效！　　普通处方

XXX医院处方笺

No.XXXXXX

自费　医保　工伤　统筹　其他

医疗证号XXXXXX　　病历号（门诊号）XXXXX

姓名　性别　男/女　年龄　岁　　年　月　日

科别　床号　地址或电话

临床诊断

Rp

纸张白色

医生

审核

调配

核对

发药

收费

¥

图 A.1　中医医院中药处方书写示例

附录 B
（资料性）
中药麻醉药品和毒性药品处方要求

B.1　中药麻醉药品处方管理

B.1.1　中药麻醉药品处方格式

开具中药麻醉药品处方应使用淡红色的麻醉药品专用处方。

麻醉药品专用处方格式由卫生主管部门规定。麻醉药品专用处方应包括患者身份证明编号，代办人姓名、身份证明编号。

B.1.2　中药麻醉药品处方的开具

具有麻醉药品处方资格的执业医师，根据临床应用指导原则，对确需使用麻醉药品的患者，应满足其合理用药需求。在医疗机构就诊的癌症疼痛患者和其他危重患者得不到麻醉药品时，患者或者其亲属可以向执业医师提出申请。具有麻醉药品处方资格的执业医师认为要求合理的，应及时为患者提供所需麻醉药品。

执业医师应使用专用处方开具麻醉药品，且不应单独开具，单张处方的最大用量应不超过 3 天常用量，连续使用不超过 7 天。

B.1.3　中药麻醉药品处方的管理

医疗机构应对麻醉药品处方进行专册登记，加强管理，麻醉药品处方宜保存 3 年备查。

B.2　医疗用毒性中药处方管理

B.2.1　毒性中药处方的开具

每次处方剂量不应超过 2 日极量。

B.2.2　处方的有效期

处方一次有效，取药后处方保存 2 年备查。

B.2.3　毒性中药的品种

毒性中药管理品种范围及用量用法简表见表 B.1。

表 B.1　毒性中药管理品种范围及用量用法

中药饮片名称	来源	用法用量	注意事项	炮制要求
生马钱子	马钱科马钱的成熟种子	0.3 ～ 0.6 g，炮制后入丸散用	不宜生用、多服、久服，孕妇禁用	将原药除去杂质，筛去灰屑，用时除去茸毛
生川乌	毛茛科植物乌头的母根	0.3 ～ 0.9 g，用时捣碎，外用适量	生品内服宜慎。不宜与贝母类、半夏、白及、白蔹、天花粉、瓜蒌类同用	除去杂质。用时捣碎
生草乌	毛茛科植物北乌头的块根	0.3 ～ 0.9 g，用时捣碎，外用适量	同生川乌	除去杂质，洗净，干燥
生附子	毛茛科植物乌头的子根的加工品	3 ～ 15 g，宜先煎，久煎	孕妇禁用。不宜与贝母类、半夏、白及、白蔹、天花粉、瓜蒌类同用	用时将原药除去杂质。洗净，取出，拭干，切片
雪上一枝蒿	毛茛科植物短柄乌头的干燥块根	内服：研末，0.062 ～ 0.125 g，或浸酒 外用：酒磨敷	有剧毒。未经炮制不宜内服。服药期间忌食生冷、豆类及牛羊肉	除去杂质
生白附子	天南星科植物独角莲的干燥块茎	外用适量，捣烂、熬膏或研末以酒调敷患处	孕妇慎用。生品内服宜慎	除去杂质
生半夏	天南星科植物半夏的块茎	3 ～ 9 g。外用适量，磨汁涂或研末以酒调敷患处	不宜与乌头类药材同用	除去杂质。用时捣碎
生天南星	天南星科植物天南星、异叶天南星和东北天南星的块茎	外用适量，研末涂患处，或捣烂以纱布包擦患处	孕妇禁用。不宜与牵牛子同用	除去杂质，洗净，干燥
生千金子	大戟科植物续随子的干燥成熟种子	1 ～ 2 g。去壳、去油用，多入丸散服。外用适量，捣烂敷患处	孕妇及体弱便溏者忌服	除去杂质，筛去泥沙，洗净，捞出，晒干，用时打碎
生巴豆	大戟科植物巴豆的干燥成熟果实	不可内服。外用研末涂患处或捣烂以纱布包擦患处	孕妇禁用。不宜与牵牛子同用。	去皮取净仁
生甘遂	戟科植物甘遂的干燥块根	0.5 ～ 1.5 g。炮制后多入丸散用	孕妇禁用。不宜与甘草同用	除去杂质，洗净，晒干
生狼毒	瑞香科植物瑞香狼毒或大戟科植物狼毒大戟、月腺大戟的根	熬膏外敷	不宜与密陀僧同用	除去杂质，洗净，晒干
生藤黄	藤黄科植物藤黄的胶质树脂	0.03 ～ 0.06 g。外用适量	内服慎用	除去杂质
天仙子	茄科植物莨菪的干燥成熟种子	0.06 ～ 0.6 g。外用适量	心脏病、心动过速、青光眼患者及孕妇忌服	除去杂质
洋金花	茄科植物白曼陀罗或毛曼陀罗的花	0.3 ～ 0.6 g，宜入丸散。亦可作卷烟分次燃吸（一次量不超过 1.5 g）。外用适量	外感及痰热咳喘、青光眼、高血压及心动过速者禁用	除去杂质
闹羊花	杜鹃花科植物羊踯躅的干燥花	0.6 ～ 1.5 g，浸酒或入丸散，外用适量，煎水洗或鲜品捣敷	不宜多服、久服。体虚者及孕妇禁用	除去杂质

（续表）

中药饮片名称	来源	用法用量	注意事项	炮制要求
斑蝥	芫青科昆虫南方大斑蝥或黄黑小斑蝥的干燥全虫	0.03 ～ 0.06 g，炮制后多入丸散。外用适量，研末或浸酒，或制成油膏涂敷患处，不宜大面积使用	本品有大毒，内服慎用，孕妇禁用	除去杂质
青娘子	芫青科昆虫绿芫青的干燥虫体	0.05 ～ 0.1 g，外用适量	体虚及孕妇忌服	除去杂质
红娘子	蝉科昆虫红娘子的干燥全虫	0.05 ～ 0.1 g，外用适量	体虚及孕妇忌服	除去杂质
蟾酥	蟾蜍科动物中华大蟾蜍或黑眶蟾蜍表皮腺体的分泌物	0.015 ～ 0.03 g，多入丸散用。外用适量	孕妇慎用	取蟾酥，捣碎，加白酒浸渍，时常搅动至呈稠膏状，干燥，粉碎。每 10kg 蟾酥，用白酒 20kg
砒石（红砒、白砒）	氧化物类矿物砷华的矿石	内服：0.03 ～ 0.075 g，入丸散用 外用：研末撒、调敷或入膏药中贴之	有大毒，用时宜慎，体虚及孕妇忌服	去净杂质，砸碎，装入砂罐内，用泥将口封严，置炉火中煅红，取出放凉，研为细粉
砒霜	砒石经升华所得到的精制品	0.009 g，入丸散用；外用适量	不能久服，口服、外用均可引起中毒	砒石升华之精制品为白色粉末
雄黄	硫化物类矿物雄黄族雄黄	0.05 ～ 0.1 g，入丸散用。外用适量，熏涂患处	内服宜慎，不可久用；孕妇禁用	取雄黄照水飞法水飞，晾干。取粉末适量，照二硫化二砷检查的方法检查，应符合规定。
水银	主要由辰砂矿炼出，少数取自自然汞	外用适量	不可内服，孕妇忌用	1. 铅制：取纯铅置容器内，加热熔化，用铁铲拨去上层黑渣，倒入水银，搅匀后倒出，放凉，研成细粉。每水银 1kg，用铅 0.4kg 2. 硫黄制：将水银与硫黄同研成末
红粉	红氧化汞	外用适量，研极细粉单用或与其他药味配成散剂或制成药捻	本品有毒，只可外用，不可内服。外用亦不宜持久用	为水银、火硝、白矾各等分混合升华而成
轻粉	氯化亚汞	内服：0.1 ～ 0.2 g/ 次，2 次 / 日，多入丸剂或装胶囊，服后漱口。外用适量，研末掺敷患处	本品有毒，不可过量；内服宜慎；孕妇禁服	粗制氯化亚汞结晶
白降丹	为氯化汞和氯化亚汞的混合结晶	外用适量	不可内服	

Foreword

Note that certain contents of this document may involve certain patents. The issuing authority of this document assumes no statutory duty to identify the patent.

The series of standards of *Requirements for Prescription, Dispensing, Delivery, Decocting and Taking of Chinese Medicine* are divided into 4 parts.

- *Part 1: Requirements for Prescription of Chinese Medicine*
- *Part 2: Requirements for Dispensing of Chinese Medicine*
- *Part 3: Requirements for Delivery of Chinese Medicine*
- *Part4: Requirements for Decocting and Taking of Chinese Medicine*

This document is the first part: *Requirements for Prescription of Chinese Medicine.*

The main drafting organizations : Jiangxi University of Chinese Medicine, Hong Kong Baptist University, Jiangxi Administration of Traditional Chinese Medicine, Shenzhen Health Development Research and Data Management Center, Macau University of Science and Technology, Health Commission of Shenzhen Municipality, Shenzhen Traditional Chinese Medicine Hospital, Shenzhen Luohu District Hospital of Traditional Chinese Medicine, Shenzhen People's Hospital, Shenzhen Institute of Standards and Technology, Shenzhen Technology University, The Fifth Medical Center of the General Hospital of the Chinese People's Liberation Army, Shenzhen Unified Standard Technology Co., Ltd, Institute of Information on Traditional Chinese Medicine of China Academy of Chinese Medical Sciences, China Traditional Chinese Medicine Holdings Co., Ltd., Inspection Office of Traditional Chinese Medicine of National Institute for Food and Drug Control, USA Hingli Health and Technology Co., Ltd., Federation of Chinese Medicine and Acupuncture Societies of Australia (FCMA), Australian Austro-Central China Medical Association, Chinese Medicine & Acupuncture Society of Australia.

The drafting organizations participants: Shenzhen Hospital of Beijing University of Chinese Medicine (Longgang), Anhui Guangyintang Traditional Chinese Medicine Co., Ltd., Dongfang Hospital of Beijing University of Chinese Medicine, Dongzhimen Hospital of Beijing University of Chinese Medicine,Bozhou Yonggang Decoction Pieces Factory Co., Ltd., Guangdong Food and Drug Vocational College, Chenghai Hospital of Traditional Chinese Medicine, HanseMerkur Center for Traditional Chinese Medicine at the University Medical Center Hamburg-Eppendorf gGmbH in Germany, Xiayuan Community Health Service Station of Suidong, Huangpu, Guangzhou, Guangzhou Jianqiao Huize Co., Ltd., Korea KyungHee University, College of Traditional Chinese Medicine of Canada, Jiangxi Jiangzhong TCM Decotion Pieces Co., Ltd., Jiangxi Institute for Drug Control, Five Branches University of California, USA Kamwo Meridian Herbs, NewYork College of Traditional Chinese Medicine, Shenzhen Hospital of Southern Medical University, The Second Affiliated Hospital of Shantou University Medical College, People's Hospital of Chenghai, Shantou, Health Center of Xinan, Chenghai, Shantou, Shantou Central Hospital,Shantou Hospital of Traditional Chinese Medicine, Shanghai University of Traditional Chinese Medicine, Shenzhen Huahui Pharmaceutical Co., Ltd., Shenzhen Institute for Drug Control, Shenzhen

Standards Alliance for Traditional Chinese Medicine Enterprises, Shenzhen Society of Traditional Chinese Medicine, Beijing Ditan Hospital of Capital Medical University, Suzhou Xinheng Automation Technology Co., Ltd, Zhongshan Hospital of Traditional Chinese Medicine.

The main drafters: Liao Liping, Lü Aiping (Hong Kong, China), Xiao Xiaohe, Wu Peikai, Li Shunmin, Zeng Qingming, Deng Xuezhi, Lan Qingshan, Ma Shuangcheng, Zhao Yonghong, Zhou Hua, Xu Ziqu, Shi Yanhong, Liu Xiwei, Chen Mingren, Zuo Zhengyun, Yang Ming, Zhou Pingsheng, Li Haiyan, Yang Jurong, Li Jinxuan, Lin Ziqiang (Australia), Yao Keqin, Kevin Chang (Australia), Zhu Lihua, Cheng Han, Zheng Jianhua (Australia) and Liang Baoshan (United States).

Drafting participants and reviewing experts(in alphabetical order of surname):Cai Benhui, Cai Chuxi, Cai Peibiao, Cai Wenwei, Cai Xiaochun, Cai Yongjiang, Chen Jianxing, Chen Jie, Chen Nie, Chen Quanhan, Chen Ruilin, Chen Siyuan, Chen Wanshan, Chen YeMeng (United States), Cheng Shiping, Cong Jialin, Cui Xinyu, Ding Yanling, Du Jianqiang, Gao Guangyin, Gao Xinyan, Gong Qianfeng, Gu Xuming, Guan Zhiyu, Guo Xiaoqiu, He Dupeng, He Lang, Hu Shiping, Hu Xiaojie, Hu Xinhua, Hua Guodong, Huang Jianfan, Huang Jukai, Huang Zhanhui, Jian Hui, Lai Manxiang, Li Jing, Li Ruijian, Li Yong, Liang Huizhou(United States), Lin Han, Lin Mingxin, Lin Shuxu, Liu Baohe, Liu Chijing (Australia), Liu ronghua, Liu Yong, Lu Haiying, Luo Guangming, Mu Fengyang, Peng Yingmei, Shi Hualan, Wang Jiabo, Wang Shuhong, Wang Weiqun, Wang Yue, Xiao Xueqing, Xu Suwen, Xu Xiaoyu, Xu Yan, Xue Chunmiao, Yang Woongmo (South Korea), Yang Xixiao, Yang Xiaohui, Yang Yinfang, Ye Nianhua, Yi Bingxue,Yu Muzhen, Yu Yawei, Yuan Xiaoning (Canada), Yuan Wenpeng, Ron Zaidman (United States), Zeng Changlong, Zha Qinglin, Zhang Delin, Zhang Jinlian, Zhang Li, Zhang Ping, Zhang Shouwen, Zhang Wenchun, Zhao Hengbo, Zhao Wenjing, Zhao Zhenping (United States), Zhu Weifeng and Zou Jiansheng.

The drafting procedure of this document complies with the *Standard Management Measures for International Organizations of the World Federation of Chinese Medicine Societies* and SCM 0001-2009 *Standards Development and Publication Work Specification* issued by WFCMS.

Introduction

Traditional Chinese medicine(TCM) is a cultural treasure of the Chinese nation. The process of TCM diagnosis and treatment starts from the patient's treatment, to the doctor's treatment based on syndrome differentiation, issuing the correct TCM prescription, and then dispensing the decoction pieces, there are corresponding key nodes in each link: How the TCM physician dispenses the prescription under the guidance of treatment based on syndrome differentiation; How to manage pharmacies and TCM prescriptions; How to check the prescription in compliance and how to adjust the prescription correctly, that is the dispensing/delivery of decoction pieces; How patients choose qualified decoction pieces for accurate formulation and reasonable decocting; How patients take Chinese medicine correctly. Each of the above links and processes is scattered without organic integration, which affects the safety and effectiveness of TCM use, damages the vital rights and interests of consumers, and further reduces the quality and reputation of TCM service.

Therefore, it is necessary to integrate the scattered TCM service links and processes into a complete system, solidified in a standard form, and build a TCM service process with traceable system, so as to reduce medical errors, improve the relationship between doctors and patients, avoid medical accidents, improve the level of medical services, ensure the safety and effectiveness of people's medication, and safeguard the legitimate rights and interests of consumers.

The purpose of the series of standards of *Requirements for Prescription, Dispensing, Delivery, Decocting and Taking of Chinese Medicine* is to integrate the service process of TCM, establish and improve the standard service system and certification system of TCM, standardize the industry behavior and the professional ethics of pharmaceutical personnel, create a safe and effective cultivation, production, circulation and drug use of TCM, promote a good atmosphere of fair, just, harmonious and scientific development of TCM trade. What's more important is that people around the world share the fruits of TCM development and make due contribution to the health of mankind.

This document is part 1, which regulates the requirements for Chinese medicine prescription. This part, which forms a seamless connection with 2, 3 and 4 parts.Prescribing is an important part of medical activities, is a very serious and rigorous behavior. And it's also the first and most important work of the entire service process.

Requirements for Prescription, Dispensing, Delivery, Decocting and Taking of Chinese Medicine
Part 1: Requirements for Prescription of Chinese Medicine

1 Scope

This document specifies the general requirement, content, and writing requirement of prescription of Chinese medicines. It regulates qualification of prescription writing, prescription of precious medicines, prescription of toxic and anesthetic medicines, and cipher prescription, etc.

This document is applicable to medical institutions and their personnel related to prescription writing, dispensing and storage.

2 Normative References

The following documents are essential to the application of this document. For dated references, only the edition cited applies. For undated references, the latest edition of the referenced document (including any amendments) applies.

GB/T 7027 *Basic Principles and Methods for Information Classifying and Coding*

GB/T 7635.1 *National Central Product Classification and Codes—Part 1:Transportable product*

GB 12904 *Bar Code for Commodity—Retail Commodity Numbering and Bar Code Marking*

GB/T 17710 *Information Technology—Security Technique Check Character Systems*

GB/T 31773-2015 *Coding Rules for Chinese Medicinal Formulae and their Codes*

GB/T 31774-2015 *Coding Rules for Chinese Medicines and their Codes*

GB/T 31775-2015 *Coding Rules for Chinese Medicines in Supply Chain Management*

ISO 18662-1 *Traditional Chinese Medicine—Vocabulary—Part 1: Chinese Materia Medica*

ISO 18662-2 *Traditional Chinese Medicine—Vocabulary—Part 2: Processing of Chinese Materia Medica*

ISO 18668-1:2016 *Coding System for Chinese Medicines—Part 1: Coding Rules for Chinese Medicines*

ISO 18668-2:2017 *Coding System for Chinese Medicines—Part 2: Codes for Decoction Pieces*

ISO 18668-3:2017 *Coding System for Chinese Medicines—Part 3: Codes for Chinese Materia Medica*

ISO 18668-4:2017 *Coding System for Chinese Medicines—Part 4: Codes for Granule Forms of Individual Medicinals for Prescriptions*

ISO 20333:2017 *Coding Rules for Chinese Medicines in Supply Chain Management*

ISO 20334:2018 *Coding System of Formulae*

3 Terms and Definitions

The following terms and definitions apply to this document.

3.1
Traditional Chinese Physician

Practitioner at institutions of medical treatment, prevention and health care, based on theories of traditional Chinese Medicines(TCM), obtaining the qualifications recognized by state-level or local health, pharmaceutical department or industry management department in accordance with laws.

3.2
Traditional Chinese Pharmacist

Practitioner at institutions of medical treatment, prevention and health care. Based on theories of Chinese materia medica, obtaining the qualifications recognized by state-level or local health, pharmaceutical department or industry management department in accordance with laws.

3.3
Doctor's Advice

Instructions given by a physician to the patient in diet, medication, and medical laboratory based on the patient's conditon and treatrment needs.

Note 1: Doctor's advice can be divided into long-term doctor's advice and temporary doctor's advice according to timeliness. The former refers to the effective time of the doctor's advice is more than 24 hours, repeated every day, and it will not be valid until the doctor indicates the stop time. The long term stand by doctor's advice is a special long-term doctor's advice that needs to be recorded in the provisional doctor's advice every time it is executed. The latter refers to the effective time within 24 hours, and it will be invalid after the completion of execution.

Note 2: According to the content of doctor's advice, it is divided into medication advice, diagnosis advice, nursing advice, entrust advice and special advice. The doctor's advice in this document refers to the medication advice, which is a medical document reviewed, allocated and checked by pharmacists and used as the medication certificate for patients.

3.4
Prescription of Chinese Medicine

Medical document issued by licensed physician for patients in the diagnosis and treatment, containing names, quantity, decocting and taking methods and other contents of the Chinese medicines and preparation of any kind of preparation, which is to be reviewed, dispensed and checked by pharmaceutical professionals of Chinese materia medica, is also a distribution voucher of medicine.

Note 1: The prescription of Chinese medicines is not only a written notice/doctor's advice, but also the basis of TCM dispensing, as well as the voucher of valuation and statistics, which has legal, technical and economic significance.

Note 2: The prescription of Chinese medicines is the written record and voucher of the doctor's syndrome differentiation and treatment, which reflects the doctor's syndrome differentiation and medication requirements.

3.5
Cipher Prescription

Regular prescriptions of medical institutions negotiated by physicians and pharmacists based on the needs of treatment, approved by the medical institutions, aiming to deal with common clinical problems with a set of fixed medicines.

3.6
Syndrome Differentiation and Treatment

According to the symptoms and signs of patients, physician summarize and judge a certain disease by analysing, synthesizing and distinguishing the etiology, nature, location and the relationship between pathogenic qi and healthy qi, and determine the corresponding treatment methods.

Note 1: The diagnosis of diseases based on syndrome differentiation is the special content of TCM diagnosis. It is the main basis of principles, methods, formulas, medicines in TCM, the basic principle of TCM for understanding and treating diseases, a special way of studying and treating diseases in TCM, and one of the basic characteristics of TCM.

Note 2: Syndrome is a pathological summary of a certain stage in the course of disease development. It includes disease location, etiology, nature and the relationship between pathogenic qi and healthy qi. It reflects the nature of pathological changes at a certain stage in the development of the disease. Therefore, it is more comprehensive, deeper and more correct than the symptoms to reveal the nature of the disease, such as hyperactivity of liver Yang and dampness-heat pouring downward. Another concept to be clear about is "symptoms", such as fever, headache, yellow coating and rapid pulse.

Note 3: Syndrome differentiation is to summarize and judge the data, symptoms and signs collected by the four diagnostic methods (inspection, auscultation and olfaction, inquiry, pulse taking and palpation) as a kind of syndrome by analyzing, synthesizing and differentiating the etiology, nature, location and the relationship between pathogenic qi and healthy qi.

Note 4: Treatment is to determine the corresponding treatment methods according to the results of syndrome differentiation. In treating diseases, TCM physician focus first on the syndrome, not on the differences and similarities of diseases. Therefore, different syndromes of the same disease require different treatment methods; and different diseases, as long as the syndrome is the same, can be treated with the same method. This is called "different treatments for the same disease, same treatment for different diseases". This principle of solving different kinds of contradictions in the course of disease development with different methods, is the spiritual essence of syndrome differentiation and treatment.

Note 5: Syndrome differentiation and treatment means that patients are identified as different syndromes of TCM according to their different symptoms and treated flexibly. It requires physicians of TCM to grasp the dynamic weather, dynamic human-being and dynamic diseases, to accurately grasp the optimal balance between the human body and heaven and earth, skilfully adjust the balance of Yin and Yang of the human body, and finally transform diseases into invisible ones by using TCM theory of "harmony between man and nature" and "syndrome differentiation and treatment". Because of the flexibility and creativity of TCM, as long as the correct mastery of syndrome differentiation and treatment, even without a clear diagnosis of the disease, these diseases could be treated. Therefore, as long as the patient has symptoms, both known and unknown diseases can be formulated for treatment and timely treatment, which is one of the biggest characteristics of TCM.

Note 6: The method of syndrome differentiation often used in clinics include eight principle syndrome differentiation, qi-blood-body fluid syndrome differentiation, visceral syndrome differentiation, six-channels syndrome differentiation, defense, qi, nutrient and blood syndrome differentiation, triple energizer syndrome differentiation, meridian syndrome differentiation. These methods have their own characteristics, in clinical diagnosis of cases, TCM physicians can flexibly integrate the above methods for syndrome differentiation and treatment.

3.7
Toxicity

Harmful effects of Chinese materia medica on the human body.

4 General Requirements

4.1 Acquisition of the Right to Prescription

After obtaining the practice qualification, doctors register in the local medical and health or industry management competent department, and they are employed by medical institutions and qualified for prescribing by such institutions.

4.2 Drawing Up of Prescription

4.2.1 Physician/doctor of Chinese Medicines should prescribe according to the principle of syndrome differentiation and treatment, specific medical needs, prevention, health care, standard of diagnosis and treatment, drug indication, pharmacological action, usage, dosage, taboo, adverse reaction and precautions, etc.

4.2.2 When prescribing narcotic drugs in an emergency state, a light red narcotic prescription should be used, and "urgent" or "critical" should be marked prominently on the upper right corner of the prescription as a reminder to enter the "Life Green Channel" of drug dispensing.

4.2.3 When prescribing pediatric emergency, doctors should weigh the first actual need to choose the colour of prescription paper: if the urgent need was greater than the safety need, the light yellow emergency prescription was used. If the need for safety is greater than the need for urgency, a light green pediatric prescription is used.

4.3 Colour of the Prescription Paper

In order to enhance the sense of visual vigilance of physicians and pharmacists, prevent medication mistakes and ensure medication safety, the prescription is divided into four colours and marked with words on the upper right corner of the prescription. Narcotic drug prescriptions are light red, emergency prescriptions are light yellow, pediatric prescriptions are light green, and general prescriptions are white.

4.4 Timeliness of the Prescription

Prescriptions should be guaranteed to be timeliness in order to ensure the timely and effective use of clinical medication.

The prescriptions of TCM are valid on that day. If the period of validity is extended in special cases, the valid period shall be marked by the prescribing physician, but the duration of the validity is not more than three days.

4.5 Revision of the Prescription

The prescription should be clear and should not be altered. If the amendment is required, the signature should be signed at the amendment and the date of revision should be marked.

4.6 Preservation and Destruction of the Prescription

The prescription should be properly preserved by the relevant medical institutions that dispense prescriptions. The duration of various prescriptions shall be kept in accordance with the requirements of the medical and health administrative department in the country or region.

The prescription should be destroyed only after it has been approved by the principal person in charge of the medical institution and after it has been sorted out, registered and put on record.

4.7 Other Requirements

The decoction pieces involved in the prescription should meet the requirements of Convention on International Trade in Endangered Species of Wild Fauna and Flora (CITES).

5 Content and Writing Requirements for Prescription of Chinese Medicine

5.1 Contents of Chinese Medicines Prescription

The contents and requirements of the preface, text and postscript of prescription writing should be standardized, which should follow the principle of safety, efficiency and economy.

—Prescription preface. The prescription preface includes the name of medical treatment, prevention or health care institution, prescription number, expense category, patient's name, sex, age and inpatient record number, department or ward and bed number, clinical diagnosis/TCM diagnosis including the disease name and syndrome type (do not write if the disease name is not clear), the date of prescribing, etc.

—Prescription text. The prescription text is marked with Rp or R (the abbreviation of Latin Recipe), and decoction pieces include it's name, dosage and usage. Chinese patent medicine prescriptions should be divided into drug name, specification, quantity, usage and dosage.

—Prescription postscript. The prescription postscript includes physician's signature and / or covered the special signature, and items with special requirements can be added according to the actual situation, such as price, drug amount, and signature and/or covered the special signature of pharmaceutical professional and technical personnel for reviewing, dispensing, checking and distributing drugs.

5.2 Requirements for Writing of Chinese Medicines Prescription

The prescription of Chinese medicines should be written in accordance with the contents of the preface, text and postscript, and should meet the following aspects:

—It should reflect the characteristic requirements of syndrome differentiation and treatment, principle-method-recipe-medicines and "Sovereign, Minister, Assistant and Guide".

—The name of the decoction pieces should be written in the official local language, and it can be noted in pinyin, or pinyin plus Latin.

—Dose of statutory dose units, with Arabia digital writing, the principle should be in "gram"(g) as a unit, "g" (unit name) followed by the numerical value.

—The special requirements for dispensing and decocting should be marked on the top right of the drug with parentheses, such as crushing, decocting first, decocting later, ect.

—If there are special requirements for producing area and Chinese crud drug processing, it should be written before the drug name.

—Choose the number of Chinese herbs per line according to the variety of the whole prescription, and in principle, it requires the horizontal upper and lower rows.

—The usage and dosage of decoction pieces should be in accordance with the provisions of the Pharmacopoeia, and there is no incompatibility of drugs in prescription. When there is an incompatibility of drugs and overdoses in a prescription, it should be signed on the top of the drug again.

—The number of decoction pieces should be used as a "dose".

—Following the number of doses, there are prescription usage and dosage includes daily dosage, dosage forms (decocting, wine-soaking, powder-baking, pill-making, capsules-filling, etc.), frequency of taking, medication methods (oral and external use, etc.), administration requirements (administered warm, administered cool, administered at draught, slow administration, administered before meal, administered after meal, administered on empty stomach, etc.).

Example: One dose per day, decocting it with 400 mL water, administered warm in the morning and evening.

—The use of decoction pieces under the administration of poison drugs and anesthetics should be strictly observed by the local relevant laws, rules and regulations.

—Prohibited or restricted use of certain decoction pieces should strictly comply with the relevant regulations of the local medical and health management departments of the country or region.

5.3 Prescription Writing Requirements for Chinese Patent Medicine

—According to the diagnosis of TCM (including disease name and syndrome type), syndrome differentiation or combination of syndrome differentiation and disease differentiation is used to select suitable Chinese patent medicine.

—The generic name of Chinese patent medicine should be approved and published by the drug supervision and administration department. The name of the decoction pieces in the hospital should be approved by the drug supervision and administration department.

—Usage and dosage should be used according to the conventional usage and dosage prescribed in the drug instructions. When the patient has a special condition and needs to exceed the dosage, the reasons should be noted and signed again.

—Tablets, pills, capsules and granules are taken as tablets, pellets, granules and bags. The ointments and cream are taken as the unit in the branches and boxes, and the solution preparations and injections are in units of branches and bottles. And the dosage should be marked.

—Each prescription should contain no more than 5 medicines. Each medicine should be arranged in rows. The medicine with strong or toxic components should avoid reusing. The Chinese patent drugs with the same function or with the same toxicity decoction pieces should not be superimposed.

—Chinese medicines injection should be prescribed alone.

—The format of the prescription can be consistent with the electronic medical record.

5.4 Writing Examples of Chinese Medicine Prescription

See Annex A for writing examples of Chinese medicine decoction pieces and Chinese patent medicine prescription.

6 Management of Prescription Rights of Chinese Medicine, the Qualification for Dispensing

6.1 Management of Prescription Right of Chinese Medicine

6.1.1 Reserve Sample for Future Reference

The signature samples and impression registration for formal and temporary prescription right of physicians should be reserved in pharmaceutical departments for future reference, which cannot be presumptuously changed by physicians without authorization. If a physician wants to change the signature pattern, he should re-register and reserve samples for future reference.

6.1.2 Prescription Right of Chinese Medicine Narcotic Drugs

According to the regulations of the health management department, medical institutions provide training and assessment on the knowledge of the use of Chinese Medicine narcotic drugs to the practitioners in this institution. Those who pass the assessment shall be granted the prescription qualification for narcotic drugs. After obtaining the qualification of prescription for Chinese Medicine narcotic drugs, a licensed practitioner may prescribe narcotic drugs in this medical institution, but he shall not prescribe the prescription for himself.

6.1.3 Modifications of Prescription

Every item of a prescription prescribed by the practitioner shall not be altered. If necessary, a straight line should be drawn on the revised content, the contents before modification should still be clearly visible, and sign the name and date again.

The prescription cannot be modified by staff majoring in decoction pieces. If the prescription needs to be modified under special circumstances such as lack of medicine or prescription errors, it should be returned to the doctor for revision and signature before dispensing.

6.1.4 Cancellation of Right to Prescription

After a doctor is ordered to suspend business and is ordered to leave the training his post to undergo training, or his practicing certificate is cancelled or revoked, his right to prescription is cancelled.

6.2 Management of Dispensing Qualification

6.2.1 Dispensing Qualification

A person who has the qualification for prescription-dispensing of the institution should obtain the professional technical qualifications for Chinese pharmacy, meet the requirements of relevant documents of health and medical industry in local country or region and be employed by the employment agency.

6.2.2 Access to Dispensing Qualification

Chinese pharmacy personnel who meet the requirements of prescription dispensing qualification can obtain the qualification of prescription dispensing only after being examined by the pharmaceutical department and approved by the institution.

Chinese pharmacy personnel who engaged in prescription review should obtain relevant professional and technical qualifications, and meet the relevant requirements of the country or region.

6.2.3 Reserve Sample for Future Reference

The signature pattern forms of Chinese pharmaceutical dispensers should be kept in the pharmacy department for reference.

6.2.4 Jurisdiction

Chinese pharmaceutical dispensers have the right to supervise and examine prescriptions, and to participate in rational clinical use of drugs. Any prescriptions that do not conform to the prescribed regulations have the right to refuse to adjust the dispensing.

7 Prescription Management of Precious Drugs

7.1 Classification and Variety of Precious Drugs

The precious drugs are divided into Class Ⅰ precious Chinese medicine and Class Ⅱ precious Chinese medicine.

The varieties of Chinese patent medicine brought into Class Ⅰ precious Chinese medicine and traditional Chinese medicinal herbs brought into Class Ⅱ precious Chinese medicine should be selected according to the "Precious Drug Management System".

7.2 Management for Prescription of Class Ⅰ Precious Chinese Medicine

The Class Ⅰ precious Chinese medicines should be managed exclusively by specially-assigned people. The prescription of Class Ⅰ precious Chinese medicines should be made out separately and stored separately.

8 Management of Cipher Prescription

8.1 Formulating principles of Cipher Prescription

The formulation principle of the cipher prescription should meet the following points:

—Necessity: there is indeed a need to treat a common clinical problem with a fixed set of drugs.

—Rationality: appropriate drugs should be chosen, i.e. they should be safe, effective, economical and appropriate.

—Stability: during pre-centralized dispensing, drugs in solid oral formulations of cipher prescription are exposed to air, and the prepared drug needs to be stored in simple packaging for a certain period of time, so the drug is required to have good stability in the air.

—Synergism: there should be no incompatibility between various drugs in the prescription, and it is better to play the role of reducing toxicity and enhancing effect.

8.2 Management of Cipher Prescription

8.2.1 Record of Cipher Prescription

Verification and recording by drug administration committee is obligatory for cipher prescription.

8.2.2 Usage of Cipher Prescription

Drugs and Chinese medicines decoction pieces prepared in accordance with the cipher prescription shall not be labelled with the name or code name of patent medicine, cipher prescription, including in medical records, should be written with the names of the specific drugs that make up the prescription. The cipher prescription shall be written in accordance with the format of Chinese medicines decoction pieces prescription.

Cipher prescription does not limit physician's flexible use of drugs, drugs may be added on the basis of the cipher prescription according to the needs of the condition, but can not reduce drugs in the cipher prescription.

8.2.3 Requirements for Instruments in Dispensing Room of Cipher Prescription

Dispensing room for cipher prescription should be equipped with instruments for modifying temperature and dampness, equipment for purification or sterilized working platform. Dispensing room should be sterilized on regular basis to ensure a neat, uncontaminated working environment with cautions of insect and dust prevention. All dispensing tools need to be sterilized on regular basis for prevention of drug contamination. The package materials that contact drugs directly should be qualified in accordance with national related stipulations.

8.2.4 Records of Dispensing Cipher Prescription in Batches

Dispensing cipher prescription in batches should be recorded involving dispensing date, commodity name, standard, originally-packaging factory, batch number, validity period of medicines in prescription, quantity of original-package drugs, number of dispensing drugs, and signatures of people in charge of dispensing and rechecking.

A label recording common names, standard, quantity, manufacturing factory, batch number and validity date of drugs within prescription is supposed to be shown on package.

8.2.5 Usage of Dismounted Drugs in Dispensing Cipher Prescription

—Dismounted drugs for dispensing cipher prescription should be used based on classifications and batches, and the date of retail should be recorded.

—Dismounted drugs are supposed to be stored with original package. If there are alternative storing containers, the quality of which should meet standard for storing drugs. Furthermore, labels involving common name, standard, manufacturing factory, batch number and validity date are required.

—Regular examination on dismounted drugs is necessary, timely disposal of unqualified products, such as contaminated drugs, deteriorated drugs and invalidated drugs is necessary, too.

9 Prescription Requirements for Narcotic Drugs and Toxic Drugs

The requirements for narcotic drugs and toxic drugs prescription should be strictly in accordance with the corresponding regulations of the health management departments of local country and region and it can also be implemented according to Annex B.

Annex A
(Normative)
Prescription Patterns and Writing Examples of Chinese Medicine in Chinese Medicine Hospitals

Writing examples of Chinese medicine prescription and Chinese patent medicine in Chinese medicine hospital are shown in Figure A.1 and Figure A.2.

<table>
<tr><td colspan="8">XXX hospital

Clinic square

Expense: medical insurance self-expense NO: 000001
Department: department of encephalopathy Nov. 25, 2009</td></tr>
<tr><td rowspan="2">Name</td><td rowspan="2" colspan="2">Yu ××</td><td>Gender</td><td>M/F</td><td>Age</td><td colspan="2">63</td></tr>
<tr><td>Outpatient record number</td><td colspan="4">2669883</td></tr>
<tr><td colspan="3">Address</td><td colspan="5">No. 15, Liulitun, Chaoyang district</td></tr>
<tr><td colspan="3">Clinical diagnosis and syndrome type</td><td colspan="5">Stroke, qi deficiency and blood stasis type</td></tr>
<tr><td colspan="8">RP: Huangqi20 g Danggui15 g Chishao10 g Chuanxiong10 g
Dilong10 g Taoren10 g Honghua10 g
Decoction 400 mL with 5 doses of water per day

Take warm fasting twice in the morning and evening</td></tr>
<tr><td colspan="2">Doctor</td><td colspan="2">Wang××</td><td colspan="2">Cost of medicine
And receipt stamp</td><td colspan="2">￥37.5</td></tr>
<tr><td>Audit</td><td>Liu××</td><td>Allocate</td><td>Li××</td><td>Check</td><td>Zhang××</td><td>Drugs</td><td>Zhao××</td></tr>
<tr><td colspan="8">Note: 1. This prescription is valid within the day
2. Please check the name, specification and quantity of the medicine when you take it
3. Reasons for extending prescription dosage: chronic senile disease other than other chronic diseases</td></tr>
</table>

Figure A.1 Writing Examples of Chinese Medicine Prescription in Chinese Medicine Hospital

XXX hospital

Clinic square

Fee: public fee NO: 000001
Department: lung disease department March 25, 2010

<table>
<tr><td rowspan="2">Name</td><td rowspan="2">Zhang ××</td><td>Gender</td><td>M/F</td><td>Age</td><td>35</td></tr>
<tr><td>Outpatient record number</td><td colspan="3">2675458</td></tr>
<tr><td colspan="2">Address</td><td colspan="4">No. 18, Happy village, Dongcheng district, Beijing</td></tr>
<tr><td colspan="2">Clinical diagnosis and syndrome type</td><td colspan="4">Cold, wind and heat type</td></tr>
</table>

RP：

Yinqiao piece 18pills×2 bags
2 pills 3 times/day oral

Doctor	Zhou××	Cost of medicine And receipt stamp	¥1.8

Audit	Wu××	Allocate	He××	Check	Sun××	Drugs	Zheng××

Note: 1. This prescription is valid for 2 days
2. Please check the name, specification and quantity of the medicine when you take it
3. Reasons for extending prescription dosage: chronic senile disease other than other chronic diseases

Figure A.2 Writing Examples of Chinese Patent Medicine in Chinese Medicine Hospital

Annex B
(Information)
Requirements for Prescription of TCM Narcotic Drugs and Toxic Drugs

B.1 Prescription Management of TCM Narcotic Drugs

B.1.1 Prescription Format for Narcotic Drugs of TCM

The prescription for narcotic drugs of TCM should use light red narcotic prescriptions.

The format of special prescriptions for narcotic drugs shall be prescribed by the competent department of health. The prescriptions of narcotic drugs should include patients' ID numbers, agent names and ID numbers.

B.1.2 Drawing Up for Prescription of Narcotic Drugs of Chinese Medicine

Medical practitioners who are qualified to prescribe narcotic drugs shall, in accordance with the guiding principles of clinical application, treat patients who are in genuine need of using narcotic drugs, the need for rational use of drugs should be met. When patients with cancer pain and other critical patients in medical institutions do not have access to narcotic drugs, *the patients* or his relatives may apply to a medical practitioner. If a medical practitioner who is qualified as a prescription for narcotic drugs thinks that the requirements are reasonable, he shall provide *the patients* with the required narcotic drugs in a timely manner.

Practicing physicians should use special prescriptions to prescribe narcotic drugs. Narcotic drugs should not be prescribed separately, and the maximum amount of the single prescription shall be no more than 3 days and the continuous use shall not exceed 7 days .

B.1.3 Management of Prescriptions of Narcotic Drugs in Chinese Medicine

The medical institutions shall register the prescriptions of narcotic drugs and strengthen the management. The prescription of narcotic drugs should be kept for 3 years for future reference.

B.2 Prescription Management for Toxic Chinese Medicine for Medical Use

B.2.1 Issue of the Prescription of Toxic Chinese Medicine

The dosage of each prescription should not exceed the two-day maximum.

B.2.2 Period of Validity of the Prescription

The prescription is effective for only one time, and the prescription is kept for two years for future reference after taking medicine.

B.2.3 Varieties of Toxic Chinese Medicine

The scope and usage of toxic Chinese medicine management varieties specified are shown in Table B.1 as a reference.

Table B.1 Scope, Dosage and Usage of Toxic Chinese Medicine

The Name of Decoction Pieces	Source	Usage	Matters Needing Attention	Processing Requirements
Strychni Semen	The dried seed of *Strychnos nuxvomica* L.(Loganiaceae)	0.3~0.6 g. After processing into the powder or pills	Should not be used raw, overdoesd or take long-term. Pregnant women are prohibited	Remove impurities from the medicine, sift away the dust, and remove the fine hair when used
Aconiti Radix	The mother root of *Aconitum carmichaelii* Debx. (Ranunculaceae)	0.3~0.9 g, mash, for external use the moderate amount is needed	Take raw with caution. It is not suitable to be used with Fritillaria Bulbus, Pinelliae Rhizom, Bletillae Rhizoma, Ampelopsis Radix, Trichosanthis Radix, Trichosanthis Fructus	Removal of impurities, mash when used
Aconiti Kusnezoffii Radix	The tuberous root of *Aconitum kusnezoffii* Reichb. (Ranunculaceae)	0.3~0.9 g, mash, for external use the moderate amount is needed	Same as Aconiti Radix	Removal of impurities, wash clean and dry
Aconiti Lateralis Radix Praeparata	The processing product of the roots of *Aconitum carmichaelii* Debx. (Ranunculaceae)	3~15 g, better to decocted early and decocted for a long time	Pregnant women are prohibited.It is not suitable to be used with Fritillaria Bulbus, Pinelliae Rhizom, Bletillae Rhizoma, Ampelopsis Radix, Trichosanthis Radix, Trichosanthis Fructus	Remove impurities from the original medicine when used. Wash, remove, dry and cut into slices

(Continuation Table)

The Name of Decoction Pieces	Source	Usage	Matters Needing Attention	Processing Requirements
Xueshangyizhihao	The dry tuberous root of the tuberculous bulb of the family ranunculaceae	For oral administration: grind to powder, 0.062~0.125 g, or vinize. For external use: rubbing the wine	Toxic. Not to be taken orally without processing. Avoid eating raw, cold, beans, beef and mutton during taking medicine	Removal of impurities
Typhonii Rhizoma	The dried tuberous rhizome of *Typhonium gigantum* Engl. (Araceae)	For external use the moderate amount is needed. Mash, boil, paste or grind the affected area with wine	Pregnant women should use with caution. Take raw with caution	Removal of impurities
Pinelliae Rhizoma	The dried tuberous rhizome of *Pinellia ternate* (Thunb.) Breit. (Araceae)	3~9 g. For external use the moderate amount is needed. Apply or grind to the affected area with wine	It is not suitable to be used with Aconite	Removal of impurities, mash when used
Arisaematis Rhizoma	The dried tuberous rhizome of *Arisaema erubescens* (Wall.) Schott or *Arisaema heterophyllum* Bl. (Araceae)	For external use the moderate amount is needed. Grind and smear the affected area, or mash and wipe the affected area with gauze	Pregnant women are prohibited. Not to be used with Pharbitidis Semen	Removal of impurities, wash clean and dry
Euphorbiae Semen	The dried and mature seeds of *Euphorbia lathyris* L. (Euphorbiaceae)	1~2 g. Remove the shell and oil, usually put into pills or powder. For external use: Apply adequate amount to the affected area	Pregnant women,the infirms and loose stools should not take	Removal of impurities, sift away the sediment, wash it, remove it, dry it, and smash it when needed
Crotonis Fructus	The dried mature fruit of *Croton tiglium* L. (Euphorbiaceae)	Don't take it orally. For external use: Apply to the affected area or mash it with gauze	Pregnant women are prohibited. Not to be used with Pharbitidis Semen	Peel and remove kernel
Kansui Radix	The dried tuberous root of *Euphorbia kansui* T. N. Liou ex T. P. Wang (Euphorbiaceae)	0.5~1.5 g. After processing into the powder or pills	Pregnant women are prohibited. Not to be used with Glycyrrhizae Radix et Rhizoma	Removal of impurities, wash clean and dry

(Continuation Table)

The Name of Decoction Pieces	Source	Usage	Matters Needing Attention	Processing Requirements
Euphoriae Ebracteolata Radix	The dried root of *Stellera chamaejasme* L. (Thymelaeaceae)	Boil to make a cream for external use	Not to be used with the Lithargyrum	Removal of impurities, wash clean and dry
Shengtenghuang	A gelatinous resin of cany yellow	0.03~0.06 g. For external use the moderate amount is needed	Oral administration should be careful	Removal of impurities
Hyosyami Semen	The dried mature seed of *Hyoscyamus niger* L. (Solanaceaea)	0.06~0.6 g. For external use the moderate amount is needed	Patients with heart disease, tachycardia, glaucoma and pregnant women should not take medicine	Removal of impurities
Daturae Flos	The dried flower of *Datura metel* L., *Datura inoxia* Mill. (Solanaceae)	0.3~0.6 g, suitable for pill or powder. It can also be used to separate cigarettes (less than 1.5 g at a time). For external use the moderate amount is needed	It is prohibited for patients with exogenous cough and asthma, phlegm-heat cough and asthma, glaucoma, hypertension and tachycardia	Removal of impurities
Rhododendri Mollis Flos	The dried flower of *Rhododendron molle* G. Don. (Ericaceae)	0.6~1.5 g. For oral administration: soaked in wine or take in pills. For external use: decocted and washed or mashed fresh and applied	Don't take too much or too long. It is prohibited for the infirms and pregnant women	Removal of impurities
Mylabris	The dried body of *Mylabris phalerata* Pallas or *Mylabris cichorii* L. (Meloidae)	0.03~0.06 g, after processing, usually put into pills or powder. External use appropriate amount, grind or dip wine, or make an oil paste to apply affected areas. Not suitable for large area use	This product has big poison. Oral administration should be careful. Pregnant women are forbidden	Removal of impurities
Qingniangzi	The dried body of the coriolaceae insect	0.05~0.1 g. For external use the moderate amount is needed	The infirms and pregnant women are forbidden	Removal of impurities
Hongniangzi	The dry whole of the red maiden of cicada family	0.05~0.1 g. For external use the moderate amount is needed	The infirms and pregnant women are forbidden	Removal of impurities

(Continuation Table)

The Name of Decoction Pieces	Source	Usage	Matters Needing Attention	Processing Requirements
Bufonis Venenum	The dried secretions of *Bufo bufo gargarizans* Cantor or *Bufo melanostictus* Schneider (Bufonidae)	0.015~0.03 g, mostly used in pill or powder. For external use the moderate amount is needed	Pregnant women should be careful	Take Bufonis Venenum, mash, add white wine to soak, stir to a thick paste, dry, crushing. For every 10 kg of Bufonis Venenum, 20 kg of white wine
Pishi(Hongpi、Baipi)	An ore of arsenic, an oxide mineral	For oral administration: 0.03~0.075 g, for powder application. For external use: grind the powder, apply or paste into the paste	This product has big poison. Use should be careful. The infirms and pregnant women are forbidden	Remove impurities, break them up, put them in a sand can, seal the mouth with mud, put them in the fire, calcined them red, take out and cool them, grind them into fine powder
White arsenic	Arsenicite is refined from sublimation	For oral administration: 0.009 g, for powder application. For external use the moderate amount is needed	Don't take long time, oral and external use can cause poisoning	The refined products of arsenite sublimation are white powder
Realgar	The mineral realgar	0.05~0.1 g, for powder or pill application. Apply proper amount to the affected area for external use	Oral administration should be careful, don't take long time. Pregnant women are forbidden	Take realgar, grind in water and dry. Appropriate amount of powder shall be taken and inspected according to the method of that of arsenic disulfide
Hydrargyrum	Mainly from cinnabar ore, a few from natural mercury	For external use the moderate amount is needed	Do not take orally. Pregnant women avoid using	1. From Lead: take pure lead and put it in a container, heat it up and melt it. Remove the black residue from the upper layer with an iron shovel. Pour in the mercury. 1 kg of mercury, use 0.4 kg of lead 2. From sulfur: grinds mercury and sulfur into powder

(Continuation Table)

The Name of Decoction Pieces	Source	Usage	Matters Needing Attention	Processing Requirements
Hydrargyri Oxydum Rubrum	Hydrargyri oxidum rubrum	For external use the moderate amount is needed, grind extremely fine powder to use alone or mix with other medicine taste into dispersing agent or make medicine twist	This product is poisonous, only for external use, not for orally. External use is not sustainable	From mercury, tint, alum mixed and sublimation
Calomelas	Mercury chloride	For oral administration: 0.1~0.2 g each time, twice a day. Mostly used in pills or capsules, and gargle after taking. For external use, amount is needed, grind and apply to affected areas	This product is toxic, not excessive. Oral administration should be careful. Pregnant women are forbidden	A crude mercuric chloride crystal
Baijiangdan	The mixed crystallization of mercuric chloride and mercuric chloride	For external use the moderate amount is needed	Do not take orally	